Fast Forward

A Comprehensive Guide to Fasting for Weight Loss

Alexandra Wells

Chapter 1: Understanding Fasting

- Introduction to fasting: What it is and its historical and cultural significance.

- Exploring different types of fasting: intermittent fasting, water fasting, juice fasting, etc.

- How fasting affects the body: physiological changes, hormonal responses, and metabolic benefits.

Chapter 2: Getting Started with Fasting

- Preparing for a fast: mental and physical readiness, setting realistic goals.

- Choosing the right fasting method for you: considerations based on lifestyle, health status, and personal preferences.

- Planning your fasting schedule: establishing a routine and maintaining consistency.

Chapter 3: The Science of Weight Loss through Fasting

- Breaking down fat loss: how fasting promotes fat burning and preserves lean muscle mass.

- Understanding calorie restriction vs. fasting: why fasting may offer unique advantages for weight loss.

- Exploring the role of hormones: insulin, ghrelin, leptin, and their impact on appetite and metabolism during fasting.

Chapter 4: Maximizing Results with Fasting

- Incorporating exercise: optimizing workouts for fasting periods and enhancing fat loss.

- Meal planning and nutrient timing: strategies for nourishing your body during eating windows and breaking fasts healthily.

- Managing hunger and cravings: practical tips for staying on track and overcoming common challenges.

Chapter 5: Fasting for Long-Term Success

- Sustainability and maintenance: integrating fasting into a balanced lifestyle for lasting results.

- Monitoring progress: tracking weight loss, body composition changes, and other health markers.

- Addressing concerns and misconceptions: dispelling myths and understanding the safety of fasting for weight loss.

Chapter 6: Overcoming Plateaus and Challenges

- Dealing with weight loss plateaus: troubleshooting strategies to kickstart progress.

- Handling social situations and peer pressure: navigating social gatherings and dining out while fasting.

- Coping with emotional eating: identifying triggers and developing healthy coping mechanisms.

Chapter 7: Fasting for Health and Wellness Beyond Weight Loss

- Exploring additional health benefits: improved insulin sensitivity, cognitive function, and longevity.

- Fasting for disease prevention and management: potential benefits for conditions like diabetes, cardiovascular disease, and inflammation.

- Incorporating mindfulness and self-care: cultivating a holistic approach to health and well-being through fasting.

Chapter 8: FAQs and Common Concerns

- Answering common questions about fasting: safety, sustainability, and potential side effects.

- Addressing concerns about muscle loss, metabolic rate, and nutrient deficiencies.

- Providing practical advice for troubleshooting challenges and optimizing fasting protocols.

Appendix:

- Sample fasting schedules and meal plans.

Introduction

"Fast Forward" offers a comprehensive yet accessible guide to using fasting as a tool for weight loss and overall health improvement. Whether you're a beginner looking to kickstart your weight loss journey or an experienced faster seeking to optimize your results, this book provides the knowledge, strategies, and support you need to succeed.

Chapter 1: Understanding Fasting

Fasting, an ancient practice spanning centuries and cultures, holds a profound significance beyond mere deprivation of sustenance. It embodies a deliberate act of abstaining from food or specific nutrients for a defined period, serving as a conduit for spiritual reflection, physical rejuvenation, and health optimization. As we embark on a journey to comprehend the intricacies of fasting, we delve into its historical tapestry, the diverse cultural manifestations, and the profound physiological transformations it instigates within the human body.

Introduction to Fasting:

Fasting transcends the boundaries of time and space, weaving its threads through the fabric of human existence. From the ancient rituals of hunter-gatherer societies to the disciplined practices of ascetics and monks, fasting has been interwoven with the narrative of humanity's quest for spiritual enlightenment and physical purification. In our modern context, fasting has evolved beyond its religious and cultural roots to emerge as a potent tool for health enhancement and weight management.

Historical and Cultural Significance:

The annals of history are replete with tales of fasting's prominence in various civilizations and belief systems. From the ritualistic fasts of ancient Egyptians to the solemn observance of Lent in Christianity, abstaining from food has been synonymous with rituals of purification, penance, and self-discipline. Across diverse cultures and epochs, fasting has served as a conduit for spiritual communion, a rite of passage marking transitions in life, and a symbol of resilience in the face of adversity.

Exploring Different Types of Fasting:

Fasting comes in various forms, each with its own set of rules and benefits. Common types of fasting include:

- **Intermittent Fasting (IF):** Cycling between periods of eating and fasting, typically on a daily or weekly basis.

- **Water Fasting:** Consuming only water for a set period, ranging from 24 hours to several days.

- **Juice Fasting:** Consuming only fruit or vegetable juices, often for a shorter duration than water fasting.

- **Extended Fasting:** Fasting for more extended periods, usually lasting beyond 24 hours, up to several days or weeks.

Each fasting method offers unique advantages and challenges, and choosing the right approach depends on individual goals, preferences, and health considerations.

How Fasting Affects the Body:

Fasting triggers a cascade of physiological changes in the body, driven by metabolic adaptations to food deprivation. These changes include:

- **Decreased Insulin Levels:** With no food intake, insulin levels drop, allowing the body to switch from glucose to fat as its primary fuel source.

- **Increased Autophagy:** Fasting stimulates autophagy, a cellular cleansing process that removes damaged components and promotes cellular repair and regeneration.

- **Enhanced Ketone Production**: Extended fasting leads to the production of ketone bodies, which provide energy to the brain and other tissues during periods of low carbohydrate availability.

- **Hormonal Regulation**: Fasting affects hormone levels, including growth hormone, cortisol, ghrelin, and leptin, which play crucial roles in appetite regulation, metabolism, and fat breakdown.

Understanding these physiological responses to fasting is essential for harnessing its potential benefits for weight loss and overall health.

In the following chapters, we will delve deeper into the practical aspects of fasting, including how to get started, maximizing results, overcoming challenges, and incorporating fasting into a sustainable lifestyle for long-term success. Whether you're new to fasting or seeking to deepen your understanding, this guide will equip you with the knowledge and tools to embark on a successful fasting journey.

Chapter 2: Getting Started with Fasting

Embarking on a fasting journey is akin to setting sail on uncharted waters, where the horizon stretches endlessly before you, beckoning with promises of health, vitality, and self-discovery. In this chapter, we shall embark upon a comprehensive exploration of the intricacies involved in initiating and sustaining a fasting practice, delving deep into the nuances of preparation, selection, and planning that lay the foundation for a successful fasting journey.

Preparing for a Fast:

Before you take the plunge into the abyss of dietary restraint, it is imperative to fortify your resolve with a steadfast commitment to your health and well-being. Prepare yourself mentally, emotionally, and spiritually for the challenges and triumphs that lie ahead, cultivating a mindset of resilience, determination, and self-awareness. Reflect deeply on your motivations for undertaking this journey, acknowledging the multifaceted dimensions of your aspirations, whether they be rooted in weight loss, metabolic optimization, or spiritual enlightenment.

Assemble the tools and resources necessary to support you on your fasting odyssey, including informational materials, supportive communities, and professional guidance if needed. Educate yourself about the physiological mechanisms underlying fasting, familiarizing yourself with the metabolic adaptations, hormonal fluctuations, and psychological adjustments that accompany prolonged periods of dietary restriction. Arm yourself with knowledge, for it shall serve as your guiding light amidst the darkness of uncertainty and doubt.

Choosing the Right Fasting Method for You:

With a firm foundation of readiness and preparation, it is time to embark upon the quest for the fasting methodology that best suits your individual needs and preferences. Survey the vast landscape of fasting practices, from the structured frameworks of intermittent fasting to the rigorous discipline of extended water fasts, each offering its unique blend of benefits and challenges.

Consider your lifestyle, dietary habits, and health status when selecting a fasting protocol that resonates with your personal goals and values. Consult with healthcare professionals or qualified practitioners if necessary, seeking guidance tailored to your specific circumstances and objectives. Experiment with different fasting modalities, exploring the diverse array of options available to you, and remain open-minded and flexible in your approach as you navigate the labyrinthine corridors of dietary experimentation.

Planning Your Fasting Schedule:

As the architect of your fasting journey, you hold the power to design a schedule that aligns harmoniously with your daily rhythm and routine. Map out your fasting periods and eating windows with precision and foresight, taking into account the demands of your work, social engagements, and personal commitments. Strive for consistency and sustainability in your fasting regimen, establishing a cadence that promotes adherence and efficacy while minimizing disruptions to your lifestyle and well-being.

Experiment with different fasting durations and meal timings, paying close attention to the subtle nuances of hunger, satiety, and energy levels that accompany each variation. Keep detailed records of your experiences and observations, documenting your progress and insights along the way. Embrace the journey with an attitude of curiosity and experimentation, viewing each fasting cycle as an opportunity for growth, learning, and self-discovery.

As you embark upon the precipice of your fasting journey, remember that the path ahead may be fraught with challenges and obstacles, but it is also adorned with moments of triumph, revelation, and transformation. Trust in your inner resilience and strength, drawing upon the reservoirs of courage and determination that lie within you. Embrace the uncertainty of the unknown with open arms, for it is within the crucible of adversity that the fires of resilience are forged. In the chapters that follow, we shall delve deeper into the mysteries of fasting, unraveling the secrets of weight loss, metabolic optimization, and holistic well-being. Prepare yourself for the epic adventure that lies ahead, as you embark upon a journey of self-discovery and empowerment through the transformative power of fasting.

Chapter 3: The Science of Weight Loss through Fasting: A Deep Dive into Metabolic Mechanics and Hormonal Harmony

In the labyrinthine landscape of weight loss strategies, fasting stands as a beacon of hope, illuminating the path towards sustainable fat loss and metabolic rejuvenation. As we embark on a journey into the intricate workings of fasting-induced weight loss, we peel back the layers of biological complexity to reveal the inner workings of the body's metabolic machinery and hormonal orchestration. Prepare to delve deep into the recesses of cellular metabolism and endocrine regulation as we unravel the mysteries of fasting's transformative power.

Breaking Down Fat Loss:

The saga of weight loss begins with the epic tale of fat metabolism, wherein adipose tissue serves as both fortress and fuel depot in the body's ceaseless battle against the bulge. During fasting, the body undergoes a profound metabolic shift, transitioning from a state of glucose-dependent energy production to one characterized by the utilization of stored fat as the primary fuel source. As glycogen stores are depleted and insulin levels decline, adipose tissue lipolysis is unleashed, liberating fatty acids into the bloodstream to be oxidized for energy production.

This process of fat oxidation forms the cornerstone of fasting-induced weight loss, as the body taps into its vast reservoir of stored fat to meet its metabolic demands. Unlike traditional calorie-restricted diets, which often result in indiscriminate loss of both fat mass and lean muscle mass, fasting exhibits a remarkable ability to preserve lean muscle mass while targeting adipose tissue for energy expenditure. Through a delicate balance of metabolic signaling and cellular adaptation, fasting engenders a state of metabolic harmony conducive to sustainable fat loss and body recomposition.

Understanding Calorie Restriction vs. Fasting:

In the arena of weight loss methodologies, the age-old rivalry between calorie restriction and fasting reigns supreme, each vying for supremacy in the battle against the bulge. While both approaches can elicit significant reductions in body weight, they diverge in their mechanisms of action and metabolic consequences. Calorie restriction entails the reduction of overall energy intake, often achieved through the manipulation of macronutrient composition or portion sizes. While effective in the short term, calorie restriction may trigger metabolic adaptations that thwart long-term sustainability and predispose to weight regain.

Fasting, on the other hand, represents a paradigm shift in dietary strategy, focusing not on the quantity but rather the timing of food intake. By alternating between periods of eating and fasting, fasting harnesses the body's inherent metabolic flexibility to promote fat loss, enhance insulin sensitivity, and optimize metabolic health. Moreover, fasting offers a simplicity and adaptability that may render it more sustainable and conducive to long-term adherence, making it an appealing option for individuals seeking lasting weight management solutions.

Exploring the Role of Hormones:

At the nexus of fasting-induced weight loss lies the intricate interplay of hormones, acting as molecular messengers to orchestrate the body's physiological response to dietary restriction and energy deficit. Chief among these hormones is insulin, the master regulator of blood glucose levels, which wields profound influence over both energy storage and expenditure. During periods of feeding, insulin promotes the uptake and storage of glucose and fatty acids, inhibiting lipolysis and promoting fat deposition. However, during fasting, insulin levels plummet, unleashing the floodgates of lipolysis and permitting the mobilization and oxidation of stored fat for energy production.

In addition to insulin, other hormones play pivotal roles in modulating appetite, energy expenditure, and metabolic rate during fasting. Ghrelin, often hailed as the "hunger hormone," surges in response to fasting and energy deficit, signaling to the brain to stimulate appetite and increase food intake. Conversely, leptin, the "satiety hormone," acts as a counterbalance to ghrelin, signaling to the brain to reduce appetite and increase energy expenditure when energy stores are replete. By finely tuning the secretion and activity of these hormones, fasting exerts precise control over appetite regulation, facilitating a natural reduction in caloric intake without the need for external restriction or deprivation.

As we delve deeper into the labyrinthine corridors of fasting-induced weight loss, we shall uncover a wealth of insights and revelations that shed light on the mysteries of metabolic mastery and hormonal harmony. Join us on this epic voyage of discovery as we navigate the turbulent waters of fat loss and metabolic optimization, forging a path towards a leaner, healthier, and more vibrant future through the transformative power of fasting.

Chapter 4: Maximizing Results with Fasting: Strategies for Optimal Fat Loss and Metabolic Mastery

In the vast expanse of weight loss strategies, fasting emerges as a beacon of hope, promising not just a reduction in numbers on the scale, but a transformation of body and mind. As we embark on this journey towards maximizing the benefits of fasting, we delve deep into the labyrinth of scientific knowledge, psychological insights, and practical wisdom to unlock the full potential of this ancient practice. Prepare to embark on an epic odyssey as we explore the myriad strategies and tactics for achieving optimal fat loss and metabolic mastery through the art and science of fasting.

Incorporating Exercise:

Physical activity stands as a pillar of health and vitality, synergizing with fasting to amplify the effects of fat loss and metabolic optimization. But the realm of exercise is vast and varied, offering a multitude of pathways towards fitness and well-being. From the rhythmic cadence of cardiovascular exercise to the transformative power of strength training, the options are endless.

Explore the vast landscape of exercise modalities, experimenting with different routines, intensities, and durations to find what works best for you. Incorporate elements of flexibility, variety, and progression into your exercise regimen, allowing for adaptation and growth over time. Whether you prefer the solitude of a solitary run, the camaraderie of a group fitness class, or the challenge of a high-intensity interval workout, there is no shortage of ways to elevate your fitness journey.

Meal Planning and Nutrient Timing:

As the saying goes, "you are what you eat," and nowhere is this more apparent than in the realm of fasting and weight loss. While fasting creates a window of opportunity for fat burning and metabolic optimization, the manner in which you break your fast and nourish your body during eating windows can significantly impact your results.

Craft a strategic approach to meal planning and nutrient timing, focusing on nutrient-dense, whole foods that provide sustained energy and satiety. Emphasize the importance of balance and moderation in your dietary choices, incorporating a variety of macronutrients, micronutrients, and phytonutrients into your meals. Experiment with different meal timing strategies, such as intermittent fasting protocols or time-restricted eating windows, to optimize fat-burning and metabolic efficiency.

Managing Hunger and Cravings:

Hunger and cravings are inevitable companions on the journey of fasting and weight loss, but with strategic planning and mindful awareness, they can be effectively managed and mitigated. The key lies in understanding the underlying triggers and addressing them proactively through a combination of dietary strategies, lifestyle interventions, and psychological techniques.

Develop a toolkit of coping mechanisms to navigate cravings and emotional eating, such as mindfulness meditation, stress management techniques, and distraction techniques. Cultivate a sense of self-awareness and mindfulness around your eating behaviors, tuning into your body's hunger and satiety cues and honoring them with compassion and respect. Experiment with different appetite-suppressing strategies, such as consuming high-protein foods, staying hydrated, and incorporating fiber-rich foods into your meals, to promote feelings of fullness and satisfaction.

Chapter 5: Fasting for Long-Term Success: Cultivating Sustainability and Thriving Beyond the Scale

In the tapestry of weight loss journeys, fasting serves as both the warp and weft, interlacing threads of discipline, resilience, and self-discovery into a fabric of transformation. As we navigate the terrain of long-term success with fasting, we embark on a voyage of self-discovery, exploring the depths of our inner landscape and charting a course towards sustainable health and well-being. Prepare to embark on an epic odyssey as we delve deep into the nuances of fasting, uncovering the secrets to longevity, vitality, and fulfillment beyond the scale.

Sustainability and Maintenance:

The true measure of success in any weight loss journey lies not in the attainment of a specific number on the scale, but in the cultivation of sustainable habits and behaviors that support lifelong health and vitality. As we traverse the landscape of fasting, we must remain vigilant in our quest for sustainability, embracing practices that nourish not just our bodies, but our minds and spirits as well.

Cultivate a mindset of long-term sustainability, recognizing that health and well-being are lifelong pursuits that require ongoing care and attention. Shift your focus from short-term fixes to lasting lifestyle changes, adopting habits that promote balance, moderation, and self-care. Embrace the journey as a process of self-discovery and growth, celebrating your progress and learning from your setbacks along the way.

Monitoring Progress:

In the journey of fasting and weight loss, progress is not always linear, and the path to success is rarely smooth. It is essential to monitor your progress regularly, not just in terms of numbers on the scale, but also in terms of how you feel, both physically and emotionally. Keep a journal to track your experiences, recording your thoughts, feelings, and observations as you navigate the ups and downs of the fasting journey.

Pay attention to non-scale victories, such as improvements in energy levels, mood, sleep quality, and overall well-being. Celebrate your achievements, no matter how small, and use them as fuel to propel you forward on your journey towards optimal health and vitality. Remember that progress is not always visible or quantifiable, and that true transformation occurs on a deeper level, within the depths of your soul.

Addressing Concerns and Misconceptions:

As fasting gains popularity as a weight loss strategy, it is essential to address common concerns and misconceptions surrounding its safety, efficacy, and sustainability. Educate yourself about the potential benefits and risks of fasting, seeking guidance from reputable sources and healthcare professionals if needed. Be discerning in your consumption of information, recognizing that not all advice is created equal and that what works for one person may not work for another.

Dispelling myths and misconceptions about fasting requires a nuanced understanding of its physiological effects and potential limitations. While fasting can be a powerful tool for weight loss and metabolic optimization, it is not suitable for everyone, and certain individuals may need to approach it with caution or avoid it altogether. Confer with your healthcare professional before venturing on a fasting regimen, especially if you have underlying health situations or concerns about its safety.

Chapter 6: Navigating Plateaus, Overcoming Challenges, and Embracing the Journey of Fasting

In the labyrinth of weight loss journeys, plateaus and challenges emerge as formidable adversaries, testing our resolve and resilience as we navigate the twists and turns of the fasting path. Yet, it is in these moments of adversity that we discover the true depths of our strength and determination, forging a path forward towards our health and wellness aspirations. As we embark on a journey through the peaks and valleys of fasting, we uncover the strategies, insights, and lessons that empower us to overcome obstacles, transcend limitations, and embrace the transformative journey that lies before us.

Understanding Plateaus:

Plateaus are a natural part of the weight loss journey, representing periods of temporary stagnation or slowdown in progress despite continued efforts towards dietary restriction and exercise. While plateaus can be frustrating and disheartening, they often serve as valuable opportunities for introspection and recalibration, prompting us to reassess our strategies, habits, and mindset on the path to long-term success.

Explore the underlying factors that may contribute to plateaus, such as metabolic adaptation, hormonal fluctuations, and changes in energy expenditure. Consider whether external factors, such as stress, sleep disturbances, or medication use, may be influencing your progress and adjust your approach accordingly. Embrace plateaus as a natural part of the journey and trust in your ability to overcome them with patience, persistence, and strategic planning.

Strategies for Overcoming Plateaus:

Overcoming plateaus requires a multifaceted approach that addresses both the physical and psychological dimensions of weight loss. Adopt strategies to reignite fat loss and metabolic momentum, such as adjusting your fasting protocol, increasing physical activity, or incorporating new dietary strategies. Experiment with variations in meal timing, composition, and frequency to stimulate metabolic adaptation and promote continued progress.

In addition to dietary and lifestyle interventions, focus on cultivating a mindset of resilience, flexibility, and self-compassion. Practice self-reflection and mindfulness, tuning into your body's cues and honoring its needs with kindness and understanding. Celebrate your progress and accomplishments, no matter how small, and use setbacks as opportunities for growth and learning.

Embracing the Journey:

Beyond the realm of weight loss and physical transformation lies a deeper journey of self-discovery, empowerment, and personal growth. Embrace the challenges and triumphs of fasting as opportunities for learning and evolution, recognizing that true transformation occurs not just in the body, but in the mind and spirit as well.

Cultivate a sense of gratitude and appreciation for the journey, recognizing the resilience and strength that lie within you. Surround yourself with supportive communities and resources that uplift and inspire you on your path towards health and wellness. Approach each day with an open heart and a spirit of curiosity, knowing that every step forward brings you closer to realizing your full potential and living a life of vitality and fulfillment.

Chapter 7: Fasting for Health and Wellness, Beyond Weight Loss

In the quest for health and wellness, fasting emerges not only as a powerful tool for weight management but also as a holistic practice that nourishes the body, mind, and spirit. Beyond its role in promoting weight loss, fasting offers a myriad of benefits that extend far beyond the numbers on the scale, encompassing physical, mental, and emotional well-being. In this chapter, we embark on a journey through the transformative potential of fasting for health and wellness, exploring its effects on longevity, metabolic health, cognitive function, and spiritual growth.

Promoting Longevity and Anti-Aging:

Fasting has long been revered for its potential to promote longevity and delay the aging process, offering a fountain of youth that extends far beyond the realm of cosmetic enhancements. Through its effects on cellular repair, oxidative stress, and inflammation, fasting exerts profound anti-aging effects at the molecular level, rejuvenating tissues and organs and bolstering resilience against age-related diseases. The mechanisms underlying fasting-induced longevity, includes autophagy, mitochondrial biogenesis, and the activation of longevity pathways such as AMPK and SIRT1. There is scientific research supporting the role of fasting in extending lifespan and improving healthspan, from animal studies to human clinical trials, and consider how these findings may inform your own fasting practice for optimal health and vitality.

Enhancing Metabolic Health:

While weight loss is often a primary focus of fasting, its benefits extend far beyond mere changes in body composition. Fasting has been shown to improve metabolic health markers such as insulin sensitivity, blood glucose regulation, and lipid profiles, reducing the risk of metabolic syndrome, type 2 diabetes, and cardiovascular disease. Fasting resets metabolic pathways, promotes fat adaptation, and improves markers of metabolic health, and contributes to overall well-being and disease prevention.

Cognitive Function and Brain Health:

The benefits of fasting extend to the realm of cognitive function and brain health, with emerging evidence suggesting that fasting may exert neuroprotective effects and enhance cognitive performance. Fasting has been shown to stimulate the production of brain-derived neurotrophic factor (BDNF), a protein that supports neuronal growth, synaptic plasticity, and cognitive function.Explore the potential cognitive benefits of fasting, including improvements in memory, attention, and executive function, as well as protection against age-related cognitive decline and neurodegenerative diseases such as Alzheimer's and Parkinson's. Delve into the mechanisms underlying fasting-induced neuroprotection, from the reduction of oxidative stress and inflammation to the promotion of neuroplasticity and neuronal resilience.

Fasting for Disease Prevention and Management:

In the tapestry of health and wellness, fasting emerges not only as a tool for weight management or spiritual growth but also as a potent strategy for disease prevention and management. Beyond its ancient roots as a therapeutic practice, fasting holds promise as a modern-day intervention for combating a myriad of chronic diseases, from metabolic disorders to neurodegenerative conditions.

Preventing Chronic Diseases:

At the forefront of modern medicine lies the battle against chronic diseases such as obesity, type 2 diabetes, cardiovascular disease, and cancer—conditions that exact a heavy toll on global health and economic well-being. Fasting emerges as a formidable ally in this fight, offering a multifaceted approach to disease prevention that addresses underlying metabolic dysfunction, inflammation, and oxidative stress.

Fasting transformative effects on insulin sensitivity, blood glucose regulation, and lipid metabolism serves as pillars of disease prevention. Fasting plays a role in reducing risk factors for chronic diseases, from improving cholesterol profiles to lowering blood pressure and reducing markers of inflammation.

Managing Chronic Conditions:

For those already grappling with chronic diseases, fasting offers a beacon of hope, providing a complementary approach to conventional treatment modalities that addresses root causes and promotes healing from within. From type 2 diabetes to autoimmune disorders, fasting's effects on metabolic regulation, immune function, and cellular repair hold promise for improving disease outcomes and enhancing quality of life.

Fasting is a therapeutic potential that shines bright across a spectrum of chronic conditions. Fasting improves glycemic control and reduces insulin resistance in individuals with type 2 diabetes, and is able to modulate inflammatory pathways and autoimmune responses in conditions such as rheumatoid arthritis and multiple sclerosis.

Harnessing the Healing Power Within:

At its core, fasting represents a return to the innate wisdom of the body, a recognition of its inherent ability to heal, regenerate, and restore balance when given the opportunity. By creating periods of physiological rest and metabolic rejuvenation, fasting empowers the body to mobilize its innate healing mechanisms, from autophagy and apoptosis to cellular repair and regeneration.

In cellular detoxification, fasting effects on autophagy and cellular repair pathways serve as guardians of cellular health and resilience. Fasting plays a role in promoting mitochondrial biogenesis, stem cell activation, and immune system modulation, and these processes contribute to disease prevention, management, and overall well-being.

Incorporating Mindfulness and Self-Care: Nurturing the Body, Mind, and Soul

In the bustling cacophony of modern life, mindfulness and self-care emerge as beacons of tranquility and rejuvenation, offering sanctuary amidst the chaos and stress of daily existence. As we navigate the complexities of fasting and health optimization, the integration of mindfulness and self-care practices becomes paramount, fostering a deeper connection with ourselves and nurturing our holistic well-being.

Cultivating Mindfulness in Eating:

At the heart of mindful eating lies a profound awareness of the present moment, a conscious engagement with the sensory experience of food, and a deep reverence for the nourishment it provides. Incorporating mindfulness into our eating habits can transform the act of nourishing our bodies into a sacred ritual, fostering a deeper connection with food and promoting greater satisfaction and fulfillment.

Practice mindful eating techniques such as slowing down, savoring each bite, and paying attention to hunger and fullness cues, allowing for a more intuitive and satisfying relationship with food. Explore the psychological dimensions of eating, such as emotional and stress-related eating, and cultivate strategies to address them mindfully, with compassion and self-awareness.

Self-Care Practices for Well-Being:

In the hustle and bustle of daily life, self-care serves as a lifeline, offering refuge and renewal amidst the demands and pressures of modern existence. From nourishing our bodies with wholesome food to nurturing our minds with rest and relaxation, self-care practices encompass a wide spectrum of activities that promote physical, mental, and emotional well-being.

The simple act of prioritizing our own needs and desires becomes an act of radical self-love and empowerment. Explore self-care practices such as meditation, mindfulness, yoga, and journaling, each offering a unique pathway to inner peace, clarity, and self-discovery. Cultivate a toolbox of self-care strategies that resonate with your individual preferences and needs, allowing for greater resilience and balance in the face of life's challenges.

Mindful Movement and Exercise:

In the dance of mindful movement and exercise, we find liberation and joy, as the body and mind unite in a symphony of breath, movement, and presence. Incorporating mindfulness into our physical activity routines can transform exercise from a chore to a celebration, offering an opportunity to reconnect with our bodies and cultivate a deeper sense of embodied awareness.

Explore practices such as yoga, tai chi, qigong, and mindful walking. Engage in physical activity with a spirit of curiosity and exploration, tuning into the sensations of movement and breath with each step and posture. Cultivate a sense of playfulness and joy in your exercise routine, allowing for greater flexibility, adaptability, and presence in the moment.

Chapter 8: Frequently Asked Questions (FAQs) and Common Concerns

In the journey of fasting for health and wellness, it's common to encounter questions, doubts, and concerns along the way. This FAQ section aims to address some of the most common inquiries and alleviate potential worries that may arise during your fasting journey.

1. Is fasting safe for everyone?

Fasting can be safe for many people, but it's essential to consult with a healthcare professional before starting any fasting regimen, especially if you have underlying health conditions or are taking medications. Certain populations, such as pregnant or breastfeeding women, individuals with eating disorders, or those with medical conditions like diabetes, may need to approach fasting with caution or avoid it altogether.

2. Will fasting slow down my metabolism?

While short-term fasting may cause a temporary decrease in metabolic rate, studies suggest that this effect is typically minimal and reversible. In fact, some research indicates that intermittent fasting may actually increase metabolic flexibility and improve metabolic health over time.

3. What can I consume during fasting periods?

The specific guidelines for fasting can vary depending on the type of fasting protocol you're following. Generally, during fasting periods, it's best to stick to zero-calorie fluids such as water, herbal tea, black coffee, or bone broth. Avoid consuming anything with calories, as this can disrupt the physiological processes associated with fasting.

4. Will fasting cause muscle loss?

When done properly, fasting should not lead to significant muscle loss, especially if you're incorporating resistance training and adequate protein intake into your routine. In fact, fasting may help preserve lean muscle mass by stimulating the release of growth hormone and promoting cellular repair and regeneration.

5. What are the potential side effects of fasting?

Some people may experience side effects such as hunger, fatigue, headaches, or irritability, especially when first starting a fasting regimen. These symptoms are usually temporary and tend to improve as the body adapts to the fasting schedule. It's essential to listen to your body and adjust your fasting protocol as needed to minimize discomfort.

6. Can fasting help with weight loss?

Fasting can be an effective strategy for weight loss, as it can help create a calorie deficit and promote fat loss. Additionally, fasting may offer metabolic benefits that support weight loss, such as improved insulin sensitivity and increased fat oxidation. However, individual results may vary, and consistency and adherence to a healthy lifestyle are key for long-term success.

7. How do I break a fast safely?

When breaking a fast, it's essential to do so gradually and mindfully to avoid digestive discomfort or blood sugar spikes. Start with small, easily digestible meals or snacks, such as fruits, vegetables, or lean proteins, and listen to your body's hunger and fullness cues. Avoid overeating or consuming large amounts of processed or high-calorie foods immediately after fasting.

8. Can fasting help with disease prevention and management?

Emerging research suggests that fasting may offer a range of health benefits beyond weight loss, including improved metabolic health, reduced inflammation, enhanced cognitive function, and even potential benefits for disease prevention and management. However, more research is needed to fully understand the long-term effects of fasting on various health conditions.

9. Is fasting suitable for athletes or physically active individuals?

Fasting can be compatible with an active lifestyle, but it's essential to tailor your fasting protocol to your individual needs and goals. Some athletes may find that fasting enhances their performance and recovery, while others may prefer to adjust their fasting schedule around training sessions to ensure adequate fueling and recovery. Experimentation and self-awareness are key to finding the right approach for you.

10. How do I stay motivated and consistent with fasting?

Staying motivated and consistent with fasting requires finding strategies that resonate with your preferences, goals, and lifestyle. Set practical goals, track your improvement, and celebrate your accomplishments along the way. Surround yourself with support from friends, family, or online communities, and focus on the positive changes you're experiencing, both physically and mentally, as you continue on your fasting journey.

Practical Advice for Troubleshooting Challenges and Optimizing Fasting Protocols

Embarking on a fasting journey can be empowering and transformative, but it's not uncommon to encounter challenges along the way. Whether you're facing obstacles related to hunger, energy levels, or adherence to your fasting schedule, the following practical advice can help you troubleshoot common issues and optimize your fasting protocol for long-term success.

1. Begin Slowly and Gradually Increase Fasting Period:

If you're new to fasting or experiencing difficulties with longer fasting periods, consider starting with shorter fasts and gradually increasing the duration as your body adapts. Begin with intermittent fasting protocols such as the 16/8 method (16 hours fasting, 8 hours eating window) and gradually extend fasting periods as you feel more comfortable.

2. Stay Hydrated and Listen to Your Body:

Proper hydration is essential during fasting periods to support overall health and well-being. Drink plenty of water throughout the day, especially during fasting periods, to stay hydrated and help curb hunger. Listen to your body's signals and adjust your fasting schedule or fluid intake as needed to ensure you're meeting your hydration needs.

3. Focus on Nutrient-Dense Foods During Eating Windows:

When breaking your fast, prioritize nutrient-dense foods such as lean proteins, vegetables, fruits, whole grains, and healthy fats to nourish your body and support overall health. Avoid processed or high-calorie foods that may lead to energy crashes or blood sugar spikes, and aim for balanced meals that provide sustained energy throughout the day.

4. Experiment with Different Fasting Protocols:

Not all fasting protocols work the same for everyone, so don't be afraid to experiment with different fasting schedules to find what works best for you. Explore variations such as alternate-day fasting, 24-hour fasts, or modified fasting regimens to see how your body responds and adjust accordingly based on your preferences and goals.

5. Address Stress and Sleep Quality:

Stress and poor sleep can impact hunger hormones, energy levels, and overall well-being, making fasting more challenging. Prioritize stress management techniques such as meditation, deep breathing exercises, or yoga to promote relaxation and reduce stress levels. Additionally, prioritize good sleep hygiene practices to ensure restorative sleep each night.

6. Stay Flexible and Listen to Your Body:

Flexibility is key when it comes to fasting, so don't hesitate to adjust your fasting protocol based on how you're feeling on any given day. If you're feeling excessively hungry or fatigued, consider shortening your fasting window or breaking your fast early with a small, nutrient-dense meal. Remember that consistency over time is more important than rigid adherence to a specific fasting schedule.

7. Seek Support and Accountability:

Surround yourself with support from friends, family, or online communities who can offer encouragement, advice, and accountability as you navigate your fasting journey. Share your experiences, challenges, and successes with others who understand and can provide valuable insights and encouragement along the way.

8. Monitor Progress and Adjust Accordingly:

Keep track of your progress, including changes in energy levels, hunger cues, mood, and overall well-being, as you continue with your fasting protocol. Use this information to make informed adjustments to your fasting schedule, dietary choices, and lifestyle habits to optimize your fasting experience and support your health and wellness goals.

By implementing these practical strategies and staying patient and persistent, you can overcome challenges, optimize your fasting protocol, and unlock the full potential of fasting for health, vitality, and well-being. Remember that every individual is unique, so it may take some trial and error to find the approach that works best for you. Stay committed to your journey, stay curious, and stay open to the transformative power of fasting as you continue on your path to greater health and wellness.

Appendix

Sample Fasting Schedules and Meal Plans

Embarking on a fasting journey requires careful planning and consideration of your individual needs, preferences, and lifestyle. Below are sample fasting schedules and meal plans to help you get started with intermittent fasting and explore different fasting protocols.

1. 16/8 Intermittent Fasting:

- Fasting Window: 16 hours
- Eating Window: 8 hours

Sample Meal Plan:

- 12:00 PM (Noon): Break the fast with a balanced meal containing protein, healthy fats, and fiber, such as a chicken salad with mixed greens, avocado, and olive oil dressing.

- 3:00 PM: Snack on Greek yogurt with berries or a handful of nuts for sustained energy.

- 6:00 PM: Enjoy a satisfying dinner with lean protein, vegetables, and a complex carbohydrate, such as grilled salmon with roasted vegetables and quinoa.

- 8:00 PM: Close the eating window with a light snack or herbal tea to promote relaxation and prepare for fasting.

2. Alternate-Day Fasting:

- Fasting Days: Consume zero or minimal calories (e.g., up to 500 calories)

- Feeding Days: Eat normally without restriction

Sample Meal Plan (Fasting Day):

- 12:00 PM (Noon): Consume a small, low-calorie meal or snack to break the fast, such as a vegetable soup or a small salad with lean protein.
- 3:00 PM: Enjoy a light snack or beverage, such as a piece of fruit or herbal tea, to tide you over until dinner.
- 6:00 PM: Have a balanced meal containing lean protein, vegetables, and healthy fats, such as grilled chicken with steamed broccoli and a side of avocado.
- 8:00 PM: Close the feeding window with a light snack or beverage, focusing on nutrient-dense options to support overall health and well-being.

3. 24-Hour Fasting:

- Fasting Window: 24 hours
- Feeding Window: Eat normally without restriction

Sample Meal Plan:

- 6:00 PM (Previous Day): Consume a satisfying dinner with a balanced mix of protein, vegetables, healthy fats, and carbohydrates, such as a stir-fry with tofu, mixed vegetables, and brown rice.
- 6:00 PM (Next Day): Break the fast with a nutrient-dense meal to replenish energy stores and support recovery, such as grilled fish with roasted sweet potatoes and a side salad.
- 8:00 PM: Enjoy a second meal or snack if desired, focusing on whole foods and avoiding excessive calorie intake to maintain balance and support overall health.

4. Modified Fasting (5:2 Method):

- Fasting Days: Limit calorie intake to 500-600 calories

- Feeding Days: Eat normally without restriction

Sample Meal Plan (Fasting Day):

- 12:00 PM (Noon): Have a light meal or snack containing protein and vegetables, such as a vegetable omelet or a salad with grilled chicken.
- 3:00 PM: Enjoy a small, nutrient-dense snack to help manage hunger and maintain energy levels, such as Greek yogurt with berries or a handful of nuts.
- 6:00 PM: Consume a balanced meal with lean protein, vegetables, and healthy fats, such as baked fish with steamed vegetables and quinoa.
- 8:00 PM: Close the feeding window with a light snack or beverage, focusing on low-calorie options to support satiety and promote metabolic health.

Remember to adjust these sample schedules and meal plans based on your individual preferences, dietary restrictions, and lifestyle factors. Experiment with different fasting protocols, meal timings, and food choices to find what works best for you and supports your health and wellness goals. Additionally, consult with a healthcare professional before starting any fasting regimen, especially if you have underlying health conditions or are taking medications.